Ana Almeida Ribeiro

# Psychological Impact of Rheumatoid Arthritis

Ana Almeida Ribeiro

# Psychological Impact of Rheumatoid Arthritis

## An Integrated Perspective

ScienciaScripts

**Imprint**



Cover image: www.ingimage.com

This book is a translation from the original published under ISBN 978-620-6-76017-7.

Publisher:
Sciencia Scripts
is a trademark of
Dodo Books Indian Ocean Ltd. and OmniScriptum S.R.L publishing group

120 High Road, East Finchley, London, N2 9ED, United Kingdom
Str. Armeneasca 28/1, office 1, Chisinau MD-2012, Republic of Moldova, Europe
Printed at: see last page
**ISBN: 978-620-7-84829-4**

# The Psychological Impact of Rheumatoid Arthritis: An Integrated Perspective

Ana Almeida Ribeiro

Happy people remember the past with gratitude, rejoice in the present and face the future without fear.

Epicurus

Contents

## Introduction

Rheumatoid arthritis is not confined to the limits of the joints it inflames; it extends, with unavoidable weight, to the fabric of the daily lives of people with this condition. The dialog between the clinical manifestation of the disease and its impact on quality of life requires an approach that goes beyond the traditionally biomedical view. This book aims to reflect this need, offering a holistic view that contextualizes RA not only as a systemic and chronic autoimmune disease, but also as a significant challenge for health systems and society.

Although the prevalence and clinical implications of RA are well documented, there is an urgent need for a more in-depth discussion of the psychosocial repercussions that accompany the disease. This text therefore seeks to delve into the intertwined paths of pain and functional incapacity, anxiety and stress, as well as depression and reduced quality of life, revealing how these aspects converge to influence the daily lives of people with RA.

Advances in the pharmacological management of RA are undeniable and have contributed significantly to improving the quality of life of those affected. However, existing treatments go hand in hand with the imperative need for physiotherapeutic approaches and non-pharmacological therapies, which are equally crucial in the management of the disease. These approaches, together with meticulous attention to treatment adherence, make up the fabric of effective and compassionate care.

We therefore propose a journey through the RA landscape, with the intention of shedding light on the best practices and policies that can support people with RA in achieving a fulfilling life, despite the challenges that the disease may impose. Recognizing RA in all its complexity is the first step towards care that truly responds to the needs of the people who live with it.

## Chap. 1 - Rheumatoid Arthritis: An Integrated View from Challenge to Resilience

### Epidemiology of Rheumatoid Arthritis

Rheumatoid arthritis (RA) is a systemic and chronic autoimmune disease that represents a significant challenge for health systems around the world. It is characterized by inflammation of the joints, which can result in severe pain, joint deformity and progressive loss of motor function, often culminating in incapacity for work and a deterioration in quality of life.

Recent international studies estimate that RA affects between 0.5% and 1% of the adult population globally, highlighting its presence across different ethnicities and socio-economic backgrounds. This prevalence underlines the magnitude of RA as a public health problem, entailing high costs both in terms of medical treatment and loss of work productivity.

RA is also associated with an increased risk of morbidity and mortality. People with RA have a reduced life expectancy compared to the general population, partly due to the systemic complications of the disease and the impact of associated comorbidities, such as cardiovascular diseases and infections.

In Portugal, the prevalence of RA was estimated at around 0.8% in 2001, with an annual incidence of new cases of between 2 and 4 per 10,000 inhabitants. This figure highlights the relevance of RA as a persistent public health challenge in the country. The impact of RA on people's quality of life is profound, with studies pointing to a significant association between RA and mood disorders, particularly depression, which amplifies the burden of the disease.

At the forefront of RA treatment, research has focused on the efficacy and safety of new therapeutic modalities.

A detailed understanding of the epidemiology of RA is crucial for developing effective public health policies and improving intervention strategies. Continued research and a multidisciplinary approach to the treatment of RA are fundamental to improving clinical outcomes and patients' quality of life, reinforcing the importance of an integrated, evidence-informed approach to the management of this disease.

## The Psychosocial Impact of Rheumatoid Arthritis

As a chronic and debilitating condition, while the physical symptoms of RA are well known, including pain, stiffness and functional disability, it is equally important to recognize and address the profound psychological and social impacts of the disease.

Rheumatoid arthritis is not just a medical condition characterized by inflammation and pain, but a disease that carries a substantial psychosocial burden that can permeate every aspect of an individual's life. The burden of RA extends far beyond the physical symptoms, profoundly affecting quality of life, interpersonal relationships and the ability to maintain an active and productive life.

RA is marked by chronic pain, morning stiffness and inflammation of the joints, which can lead to a progressive loss of mobility and joint deformity.

Pain and functional disability are two of the most challenging aspects of rheumatoid arthritis, imposing significant barriers to performing daily activities such as dressing, cooking or even simple self-care tasks, and to engaging in social relationships

Pain in rheumatoid arthritis is persistent and often debilitating, caused by both joint inflammation and joint deterioration. The intensity of the pain can vary, influenced by factors such as the weather, physical activity and stress levels. This symptom not only limits physical mobility, but also acts as a constant reminder of the limitations imposed by the disease, affecting the person's psychological state.

The functional incapacity generated by RA is one of the main factors contributing to dependence on others, which can foster feelings of frustration and loss of personal autonomy.

The restrictions imposed by the physical symptoms of RA often trigger a cascade of emotional impacts. Many people experience feelings of anxiety and depression due to uncertainty about the progression of the disease and fear of future pain and disability. The constant worry about health can create a state of continuous alertness and tension, significantly reducing mental and emotional well-being.

Social isolation is a common consequence of RA, caused by both physical limitations and emotional decline. People may withdraw from their social networks and activities that used to bring them pleasure and satisfaction, contributing to a sense of isolation and loneliness. In addition, family relationships and friendships can be affected, as the disease imposes a new dynamic on interactions and the emotional support needed.

In addition to the physical and emotional dimensions, RA has significant economic implications. Many people find themselves unable to work due to pain and functional disability, which can lead to a loss of income and, consequently, a deterioration in living conditions. The cost of medical treatment, often long-term and intensive, also represents a considerable financial burden for people with RA and their families.

The burden of rheumatoid arthritis is multifaceted and deeply integrated into the physical, emotional, social and economic aspects of the lives of people with RA.

Anxiety and stress are common responses in people with RA, appearing both as reactions to the chronic pain and uncertainty of the disease and as exacerbators of physical symptoms.

Anxiety in patients with RA often stems from fear of the progression of the disease, the possible loss of autonomy and the changes in lifestyle that the condition may require. Constant worry about future joint deformities or the ability to maintain independence can create a persistent state of tension and vigilance.

Stress can directly aggravate inflammation, playing a significant role in RA activity. Prolonged stressful situations can not only worsen physical symptoms, but also decrease the effectiveness of the immune system, further complicating the person's state of health. Stress management therefore becomes crucial to controlling disease activity and improving quality of life.

Anxiety and stress can also compromise the effectiveness of treatment, as they can affect adherence to prescribed therapies and willingness to participate in rehabilitation or self-help activities.

Depression is a common and one of the most debilitating consequences among people with RA. The perception of deteriorating health and limited functionality can lead to a significant decrease in quality of life, affecting their emotional and social well-being. Depression not only affects mood and motivation, but can also have a negative impact on family and social relationships, work performance and the ability to maintain an active lifestyle.

People with RA face a high risk of developing depression due to chronic pain, physical limitations and uncertainty about the future. Depression can worsen the perception of pain, create barriers to effective treatment and isolate people.

Quality of life in people with RA is directly impacted by depression, which can reduce motivation to participate in recreational and social activities, decrease effectiveness at work or in daily tasks, and negatively affect personal relationships. Social isolation is both a cause and an effect of depression, creating a cycle that is difficult to break without appropriate intervention.

The treatment of depression in people with RA should include psychopharmacological therapies, where appropriate, and psychotherapies such as cognitive-behavioral therapy. Adapted exercise programs and occupational therapies can also improve autonomy and well-being, helping to break the cycle of depression. Continued education about the illness and the active involvement of people in the treatment plan are essential for increasing the sense of control and reducing depressive symptoms.

Considering the complexity of the psychosocial impacts of RA, an integrated approach that includes pain and inflammation management, along with psychological and social support, is essential. Rehabilitation programs, support groups and psychotherapeutic interventions can be instrumental in helping people with RA develop effective coping strategies, reduce stress and improve mental health. Ongoing education about the disease, both for people with RA and their families, is crucial to foster an environment of mutual support and understanding.

Recognizing and treating the psychosocial aspects of RA is just as important as managing the physical symptoms. Adopting a holistic approach to treating RA can significantly improve people's quality of life, providing them not only with physical relief, but also with emotional and psychological support. Collaboration between rheumatologists, nurses, psychologists, physiotherapists and other health professionals is vital for developing a complete care plan that addresses all aspects of this challenging condition.

## Treatment and Management of Rheumatoid Arthritis

Rheumatoid arthritis, if not managed properly, can result in significant joint deformities and loss of functionality. Effective treatment and management of RA are crucial to improving people's quality of life and minimizing the impact of the disease.

The pharmacological treatment of rheumatoid arthritis essentially aims to control inflammation, relieve pain and prevent progressive joint damage. The therapeutic approach is typically staggered, starting with less potent drugs and progressing to more advanced options according to clinical need.

### Analgesics and Non-Steroidal Anti-Inflammatory Drugs (NSAIDs)

Analgesics, particularly paracetamol, are often used for pain relief in RA patients, although their effect on inflammation is limited. NSAIDs, such as ibuprofen and diclofenac, are more effective in treating inflammation and are commonly prescribed to reduce both pain and joint swelling. However, prolonged use of NSAIDs can be associated with significant side effects, including gastrointestinal and cardiovascular problems, which requires careful monitoring.

### Corticosteroids

Corticosteroids, such as prednisolone, are potent anti-inflammatory agents used to control acute bouts of inflammation in RA. They are effective in relieving symptoms quickly and are often used for short periods to minimize long-term side effects, which can include osteoporosis, increased risk of infections and metabolic changes.

### Disease Modifying Anti-Rheumatic Drugs (DMARDs)

DMARDs are the backbone of RA treatment and are key to preventing long-term joint damage. Drugs such as methotrexate, leflunomide and sulfasalazine are often used as first-line therapy. These drugs can slow down the progression of the disease and improve quality of life, but they also require regular monitoring due to the risk of liver, kidney and hematological toxicity.

## Biological agents

For more severe cases or when patients do not respond adequately to traditional DMARDs, biological agents such as etanercept, infliximab and adalimumab, among others, are used. These drugs target specific components of the immune system involved in inflammation. Biological agents have shown high efficacy in reducing symptoms and preventing joint damage, but their high cost and the potential for serious side effects, including opportunistic infections, are important considerations.

## Therapeutic advances

As far as treatment is concerned, the evolution of therapies has been remarkable, with the introduction of Janus Kinase inhibitors and new glucocorticoid modalities and biological therapies that promise more effective management of the disease. Recent research points to the potential of targeted treatments, adjusted to the individual pathophysiology of the person, indicating an era of personalization in the treatment of RA.

**The Interrelationship of Cytokines and the Impact of Lifestyle**

The interaction of cytokines in the pathogenesis of RA has also been studied, revealing the complexity of the disease and the need for a deeper understanding of the underlying immunological mechanisms. Factors such as physical exercise and diets enriched with omega-3 show potential for mitigating the effects of RA, highlighting the importance of a multidisciplinary approach to managing the disease.

Although pharmacological treatment is fundamental in the management of rheumatoid arthritis, physiotherapeutic approaches and non-pharmacological therapies play an equally crucial role. These therapies help complement medical treatment by addressing the physical and functional aspects that affect patients' quality of life.

Specific physical exercises are essential for people with RA, as they help maintain range of motion, reduce stiffness and strengthen the muscles that support the affected joints. Exercise programs can include low-impact activities such as swimming or walking, which are effective in promoting mobility without overloading the joints. Regular practice of these activities helps to prevent functional deterioration and maintain a person's independence.

Rehabilitation in patients with RA is focused on restoring functionality, reducing pain and improving the performance of daily activities. Techniques such as hydrotherapy, which uses the properties of water to relieve pressure on joints and improve mobility, are often recommended. In addition, manual therapy, including massage and joint mobilization, can be used to relieve pain and improve movement.

Occupational therapies are vital in helping people with RA adapt to their daily limitations. These therapies involve adapting the person's living and working environment, ensuring that they can perform their tasks with minimal discomfort. Occupational therapists work on customizing everyday utensils, such as adaptive cutlery and dressing aids, to help maintain autonomy and quality of life.

Integrating these approaches is key to promoting autonomy and quality of life. Education on disease self-management and coping techniques are integral parts of treatment, allowing people to take an active role in managing their condition.

## Treatment Adherence Challenges in the Management of Rheumatoid Arthritis

Adherence to treatment is one of the biggest challenges in the management of rheumatoid arthritis, with significant implications for the effectiveness of treatment and the quality of life of people with the condition. The complexity of the therapeutic regimen, together with the psychological impact of RA, can create substantial obstacles that prevent adequate adherence.

The psychological impact of RA, including depression, anxiety and stress, can profoundly affect the ability of a person with RA to adhere to their treatment plan. Depression and anxiety can decrease motivation, while stress can interfere with the ability to effectively manage medication and health commitments. In addition, chronic pain and fatigue can make it difficult for people with RA to maintain regularity and accuracy in taking their medication.

**Barriers to membership**

There are several barriers that can influence adherence, including:

- **Complexity of the Therapeutic Regimen**: Treatment regimens with multiple medications and complicated dosage schedules can be difficult to follow.

- **Side effects**: The adverse effects of some drugs can discourage people from continuing treatment.
- **Financial costs**: The high cost of medicines, especially biological agents, is a significant barrier for many people.
- **Lack of Social Support**: The lack of a support network can decrease adherence, especially if the person with RA needs help getting to appointments or managing their medication.

**Strategies to Improve Adherence**

To overcome these barriers, various strategies can be implemented:

- **Continuing Education**: Providing understandable and up-to-date information about RA and its treatment can help people understand the importance of adherence for disease control.
- **Psychosocial support**: Support programs that address emotional and psychological well-being can improve adherence to treatment by offering coping strategies.
- **Side effect management**: Working with health professionals to adjust therapeutic regimens and minimize side effects can encourage greater adherence.

- **Regular follow-up**: Regular consultations with the healthcare team help to monitor progress and adjust treatment as necessary, as well as reinforcing the importance of adherence.

The challenges in adhering to treatment for people with RA are multifaceted and require an integrated approach that considers both clinical and psychological aspects. Improving adherence involves understanding the individual needs of each person with RA and adapting the support offered to meet those needs, thus ensuring better therapeutic results and a better quality of life.

## Chap. 2 - Mental Health Theories Applied to the Context of Rheumatoid Arthritis

Mental health plays a crucial role in the experience and clinical outcomes of people with rheumatoid arthritis. Understanding and applying mental health theories in this context allows us not only to address the physical symptoms of the disease, but also to recognize and treat its profound emotional and psychological impacts.

### Behavioral and Cognitive Theories

Behavioral and cognitive theories are extremely pertinent in understanding RA, especially when it comes to how people deal with chronic pain and disability. These theories suggest that people's thoughts and behaviors can influence the way they perceive their pain and their ability to manage the disease. Interventions based on cognitive-behavioral therapy (CBT) have been shown to be effective in reducing depression and anxiety, while also improving adherence to treatment and quality of life.

### Biopsychosocial Model

The biopsychosocial model is fundamental to understanding RA, as it recognizes the interaction between biological, psychological and social factors in health. This model suggests that RA treatment should go beyond medical interventions to include psychological and social support, which are crucial for dealing with the complexity of the disease. Integrating mental health services into primary care can facilitate this process by providing a more coordinated and holistic approach.

**Stress and Adaptation Theory**

The theory of stress and adaptation can be applied to help understand how people with RA cope with the chronic stress caused by the disease. This theory helps to explore the coping strategies that people develop to deal with the disease and its limitations. Intervention programs that teach stress management techniques, such as relaxation and problem solving, can be particularly beneficial.

**Humanism and Person-Centered Care**

The humanistic approach to RA treatment emphasizes the importance of treating each person as a unique individual with specific rights and needs. This approach supports the idea that care should be person-centered, not just disease-centered. The practice of active listening and empathy on the part of health professionals can strengthen the therapeutic relationship and improve treatment outcomes.

## Applying Hildegard Peplau's Nursing Theory to the Context of Rheumatoid Arthritis

Hildegard Peplau stood out for her focus on interpersonal relationships as a critical component of the nursing care process. In the context of RA, where physical and psychological challenges are intrinsically linked, the application of this theory can transform care, offering more integral, person-centered support.

### Peplau and AR's Interpersonal Relationship Phases

**Orientation phase:** In this initial phase, the person with RA and the nurse establish a relationship. The nurse acts as a leading figure to clarify doubts about the disease and available treatments. Creating an environment of trust is crucial for the person to feel comfortable expressing their concerns and fears related to RA.

**Identification phase:** During this phase, the person with RA begins to identify problems and challenges they face, with the help of the nurse. Together, they begin to define goals for pain management, improving mobility and optimizing quality of life. This is a time when the person is actively involved in their own care process.

**Exploration phase:** Here, the nurse helps the person with RA to explore coping strategies and adaptations needed to deal with the disease. This can include adjustments to the daily routine, relaxation techniques, and the introduction of adapted physical activities that promote joint health without causing an exacerbation of symptoms.

**Resolution phase:** In the final phase, the person with RA begins to integrate the new strategies learned and make more informed decisions about their care. The nurse continues to offer support, but encourages independence, preparing the person to manage their health more autonomously.

**Benefits of Peplau's Theory in HR Management**

The application of Interpersonal Relations Theory can significantly improve the management of RA, as it emphasizes education, emotional support and the development of personal skills to cope with the disease. This person-centered approach helps strengthen autonomy and self-efficacy, essential components for coping with a chronic condition like RA.

The application of mental health theories to the context of rheumatoid arthritis is not only an expansion of clinical understanding, but a practical necessity to address the complexity of the challenges faced by these people. The theories discussed provide a framework for developing more effective interventions and more comprehensive and empathetic care. Integrating Peplau's theory into the care of people with rheumatoid arthritis not only enriches clinical support, but also promotes a stronger therapeutic relationship, which can be fundamental in facing the physical and emotional challenges of the disease. The nurse, following this model, becomes a vital partner in the care process, helping the person with RA to navigate the complexities of treatment and adapting to life with the disease.

## Chapter 3: Psychoemotional Profiles in Rheumatoid Arthritis: An Analysis of Anxiety, Depression and Stress

### Main results

A study conducted in a hospital unit in northern Portugal revealed a notable prevalence of anxiety, depression and stress among individuals with rheumatoid arthritis. It was found that 75% of participants had moderate to high levels of anxiety, while depression affected 72.5% of respondents. On the other hand, stress was high in

57.5% of cases. This data highlights the psycho-emotional challenges faced by this population, overcoming the purely somatic obstacles of the condition.

Particularly revealingly, the study found that monthly family income was inversely related to negative psycho-emotional states, which were more prominent in participants with lower incomes. However, other sociodemographic variables, such as marital status and educational qualifications, had no significant impact on levels of anxiety, depression and stress.

**Discussion of results**

The correlation between general disease status and psycho-emotional indices highlights a critical dimension in the management of rheumatoid arthritis. General disease status explains approximately 20% of the variance observed in anxiety and depression and 10% in stress. This interconnection points to the multifactorial reality of RA, where disease management must extend beyond the physical sphere, encompassing the psycho-emotional elements that amplify the impact of the disease on people's quality of life.

By delving into these results, we recognize that RA treatment cannot be dissociated from active psychosocial intervention. Integrated care involving tailored therapeutic strategies, continuing education and robust psychological support is essential. The implementation of such measures can promote not only the improvement of physical symptoms, but also enhance the emotional and psychological well-being of those affected.

This chapter, which is part of a book, aims to broaden the discussion on the psycho-emotional dimensions of RA, challenging the academic and professional community to consider the holistic complexity of the disease. It therefore aims to foster a paradigm of care that aligns with the principles of a contemporary and empathetic clinical practice, geared towards the integral health of the person with RA.

## Chapter 4: Implications for Clinical Practice and Health Policy in Rheumatoid Arthritis

Rheumatoid arthritis is not only a clinical challenge, but also a public health problem with profound socio-economic implications. The findings presented in this book highlight the need for an integrated approach in clinical practice and health policies, which considers both the management of the disease and its psychosocial impact.

## Implications for Clinical Practice

**Integrated Pain Management:** It is imperative that treatment strategies for RA encompass not only pharmacological pain control, but also psychotherapeutic and educational interventions to deal with the consequences of chronic pain.

**Psychosocial monitoring:** Health professionals should be alert to signs of anxiety, depression and stress in people with RA, integrating regular psychosocial assessments as part of disease monitoring.

**Health Education: Health education** programs should be developed to inform people with RA about the nature of their condition, self-management strategies and the importance of adherence to treatment.

**Professional Training:** Continuing training in mental health for health professionals is essential to equip the multidisciplinary team with the necessary skills to offer holistic care.

## Public Health Policies

**Equitable Access to Treatment:** Policies should be implemented to ensure equitable access to effective treatments for RA, regardless of people's income or geographical location.

**Support for Research and Development:** Investment in research is vital for the development of new therapies and for a deeper understanding of the psychosocial aspects of RA.

**Early Intervention Programs:** Programs that promote the early detection and intervention of RA can help reduce the progression of the disease and improve long-term outcomes.

**Integration of Health Services:** Strategies that favor the integration of rheumatology, nursing, physiotherapy, psychology and occupational therapy services can facilitate more efficient, person-centered management.

The multifaceted impact of rheumatoid arthritis requires that both clinical practice and health policies adapt to meet the complex needs of those affected. The development of public health policies that emphasize prevention, education, integrated management and psychosocial support is key to improving the quality of life of people with RA.

## Conclusion

At the end of this book, the message clearly resonates that rheumatoid arthritis is an experience that transcends joint pain and inflammation. The need for approaches that integrate the various dimensions of being - physical, psychological and social - for more effective and humane care has become clear. This holistic view not only reaffirms the importance of biomedical management of the disease, but also underlines the inestimable value of a robust support network and appropriate psychosocial interventions. The role of health professionals in this context is not limited to prescribing and advising, but extends to listening, understanding and walking alongside the person with RA at every stage of their journey.

The lessons learned here highlight the importance of health policies that promote accessibility and equity in the treatment of RA, ensuring that every person, regardless of their socioeconomic status or geographical location, can enjoy quality healthcare. Strategies that promote health education, prevention and integrated disease management emerge as pillars for a more promising future in RA management.

We close this book with a look to the future, where scientific innovation and therapeutic advances will continue to be vital. However, it is imperative that all those involved in the RA journey - rheumatologists, nurses, physiotherapists, occupational therapists, psychologists, social workers, policy-makers and, above all, people with RA themselves - collaborate in a symbiosis of efforts. Constant dialogue between research and clinical practice is crucial to meeting the challenges posed by this condition.

Throughout this short book, we have tried to shed light on the less visible aspects of RA, those that are embedded in the daily lives and lives of the people who live with it. Through a discourse informed by studies, reports and recommended practices, a panorama has been outlined that goes beyond the clinical horizon and reaches the fertile ground of human experiences.

## Bibliographical references


- Bértolo, M. (2008) - How to diagnose and treat rheumatoid arthritis Taken from: http://www.cibersaude.com.br/revistas.asp?fase=R003&id_materia=3949, consulted on September 30, 2014.
- Brito, M.; Goes, L.; Costa, V.; Gurgel, M.; Alves M.; Timbó, M; Bezerra Filho, J. (2013). Burn-related suicide attempt: suicidal ideation and hopelessness. Revista Brasileira Queimaduras. 2013, 12 (1): 30-36. Taken from: http://www.rbqueimaduras.com.br/detalhe_artigo.asp?id=141, consulted on November 10, 2014.
- Brouwer, S. M., van Middendorp, H., Kraaimaat, F. W., Radstake, T. J., Joosten, I., Donders, A. T., & Evers, A. M. (2013). Immune responses to stress after stress management training in patients with rheumatoid arthritis. Arthritis Research & Therapy. 15(6). Retrieved from: http://web.b.ebscohost.com/ehost/pdfviewer/pdfviewer?vid=24&sid=ee16b3c8- f03e-46d3-9cea-55f89e63fcf2%40sessionmgr110&hid=105, accessed October 22, 2014.
- Buendgens, F. B., Blatt, C. R., Marasciulo, A. C. E., Leite, S. N., & Farias, M. R. (2013). Cost-Analysis

Study of the Treatment of Severe Rheumatoid Arthritis in a Municipality in Southern Brazil. *Cadernos De Saúde Pública.* https://doi.org/10.1590/0102-311x00013513

- Clarice Gomes e Souza, D., Almeida, A. M., & Acúrcio, F. d. A. (2015). Non-Adherence to Biological Therapy in Patients with Rheumatic Diseases in the Unified Health System in Minas Gerais, Brazil. *Cadernos De Saúde Pública.* https://doi.org/10.1590/0102-311x00169514
- Corbacho, M.I., Dapueto, J.J. (2010). Evaluation of functional capacity and quality of life in patients with rheumatoid arthritis. Rev Bras Reumatol 2010;50(1):31-43. Taken from: http://www.scielo.br/pdf/rbr/v50n1/v50n1a04.pdf, consulted on November 14, 2014.
- Coutinho, C. P. (2013). Research Methodology in Social Sciences and Humanities: theory and practice. 2nd edition. Coimbra. Almedina. 84
- Covic, T., Cumming, S., Pallant, J., Manolios, N., Emery, P., Conaghan, P., & Tennant, A. (2012). Depression and anxiety in patients with rheumatoid arthritis: prevalence rates based on a comparison of the Depression, Anxiety and Stress Scale (DASS) and the hospital, Anxiety and Depression Scale (HADS).

Taken from: http://www.biomedcentral.com/1471-244X/12/6, consulted on October 22, 2014.

- Dario, A.B., Külkamp, W., Faraco, H.C., Gevaerd, M.S., & Domenech, S.C.. (2010). Psychological changes and physical exercise in patients with rheumatoid arthritis. Motricidade, 6(3), 21-30. Retrieved from: http://www.scielo.mec.pt/scielo.php?script=sci_arttext &pid=S1646- 107X2010000300004&lng=en&tlng=en, accessed March 30, 2015.
- Deighton, C., O'Mahony, R., Tosh, J., Turner, C., & Rudolf, M. (2009). Management of Rheumatoid Arthritis: Summary of NICE Guidance. *BMJ.* https://doi.org/10.1136/bmj.b702
- DGS (2005). National Plan Against Rheumatic Diseases. Taken from: http://www.dgs.pt/outros-programas-e-projetos/paginas-de-sistema/saude-de-a-az/programa-nacional-contra-as-doencas-reumaticas.aspx, consulted on November 11, 2013. • DGS (2011). Prescription of Biological Agents in Rheumatic Diseases. Taken from: http://www.dgs.pt/directrizes-da-dgs/normas-e-circulares-normativas/norma-n0672011-de-30122011.aspx, consulted on October 22, 2014.

- DGS (2012). National Program for Rheumatic Diseases: Programmatic Guidelines. Taken from: http://www.dgs.pt/programas-de-saude-prioritarios.aspx, consulted on November 10, 2013.
- DGS (2013). Portugal: Mental Health in numbers - 2013. Taken from: http://www.dgs.pt/portal-da-estatistica-da-saude/publicacoes-estatisticas.aspx, consulted on November 10, 2013. 85
- DGS (2013). Rheumatology Hospital Referral Network. Taken from: http://www.dgs.pt/upload/membro.id/ficheiros/i006184.pdf, consulted on November 09, 2013.
- Dirik, G., & Karanci, A. (2010). Psychological distress in rheumatoid arthritis patients: an evaluation within the conservation of resources theory. Psychology & Health, 617-632.
- Duarte, C. , Simões, S. (2010). Disease activity and quality of life in patients with Rheumatoid Arthritis. Revista Referência II Série - n.º12 - Mar. 2010. Pp 35-44. Taken from: file:///C:/Users/Ana/Downloads/3.%C2%BA_Classificado.pdf, consulted on December 28, 2014.
- Fechtenbaum, M., Nam, J. L., & Emery, P. (2014). Biologics in rheumatoid arthritis: where are we going? Retrieved from:

http://web.a.ebscohost.com/ehost/pdfviewer/pdfviewer?sid=73f41158-c6df-4d7e851c-ca275fc48d44%40sessionmgr4003&vid=22&hid=4112, accessed December 28, 2014.

- Ferri (2014). Major Depression. Copyright. Pp 325-326. Retrieved from: www.clinicalkey.com, accessed November 11, 2013. A.; Bhadauria, D. (2013). Evaluation of efficacy of fluoxetine in the management of major depression and arthritis in patients of Rheumatoid Arthritis. Retrieved from: http://www.indianjrheumatol.com/article/S0973-3698(13)00106-4/fulltext, accessed November 10, 2013. 87• Kekow, J., Moots, R., Khandker, R., Melin, J., Freundlich, B., & Singh, A. (2011). Improvements in patient-reported outcomes, symptoms of depression and anxiety, and their association with clinical remission among patients with moderate-to-severe active early rheumatoid arthritis. Rheumatology (Oxford, England),50 (2), 401-409. Taken from: http://rheumatology.oxfordjournals.org/content/50/2/401.full.pdf, consulted on October 22, 2014.
- Gurgel, T. L., & Oliveira, F. d. S. (2022). Repercussions of Glucocorticoids in the Treatment of Rheumatoid Arthritis: A Review. *Educação Ciência E Saúde.* https://doi.org/10.20438/ecs.v9i1.414

- Lícia Maria Henrique da, M., Cruz, B. A., Brenol, C. V., Pereira, I. A., Fronza, L. S. R., Bértolo, M. B., Freitas, M. V. C., Silva, N. A. d., Louzada-Júnior, P., Giorgi, R. D. N., Lima, R. A. C., & Geraldo da Rocha Castelar, P. (2011). 2011 Brazilian Society of Rheumatology Consensus for the Diagnosis and Initial Evaluation of Rheumatoid Arthritis. *Brazilian Journal of Rheumatology.* https://doi.org/10.1590/s0482-50042011000300002
- Lucas, R. & Monjardino, T (2010). The State of Rheumatology in Portugal. Taken from: http://ondor.med.up.pt/uploads/pdf/ONDOR_Estado_Reumatologia_Portugal-1.pdf, consulted on November 09, 2013.
- Malysheva, O., Pierer, M., Wagner, U., & Baerwald, C. O. (2010). [Stress and rheumatoid arthritis]. Zeitschrift Für Rheumatologie, 69(6), 539-543. Retrieved from: http://search.ebscohost.com/login.aspx?direct=true&db=mdc&AN=20652573&lang =en-br&site=ehost-live
- Merlino, A. B., Schafranski, M. D., Mansani, F. P., Grace Arrielo de Castro, P., & Carolyn Maria de Geus, W. (2015). Role of Anti-CCP Antibodies in Different Autoimmune Diseases. *Brazilian Journal of Internal Medicine.* https://doi.org/10.15743/rbmi.2015.0001

- Moreira, F. F., Tartari, A. P. S., Kerppers, I. I., Mário César da Silva, P., Julik, A. D., Suckow, P. P. T., Eliane Gonçalves de Jesus, F., Massuqueto, R. R. H., & Bini, A. C. D. (2022). Ozone Treatment in Rheumatoid Arthritis: A Systematic Review. *Cadernos De Educação Saúde E Fisioterapia.* https://doi.org/10.18310/2358-8306.v9n19.a11
- Negrão, Â. S., Igor Mateus Fernandes de, O., Vieira, D. A., Lima, A. B. d., & Coelho, H. R. (2021). Physical Exercise and Rheumatoid Arthritis: Intervention Possibilities of a Training Protocol. *Research Society and Development.* https://doi.org/10.33448/rsd-v10i9.18481
- Pereira da Silva, J. (2005). Practical Rheumatology. Diagnóstico, Lda. Coimbra
- Pereira, I. A., & Pereira, R. M. R. (2004). Osteoporosis and Focal Bone Erosions in Rheumatoid Arthritis: From Pathogenesis to Treatment. *Brazilian Journal of Rheumatology.* https://doi.org/10.1590/s0482-50042004000500006
- Pereira, L. P. S., & Maia, M. d. S. (2021). Main Physiotherapeutic Approaches in the Treatment of Rheumatoid Arthritis: A Bibliographic Review. *Research Society and Development.* https://doi.org/10.33448/rsd-v10i12.20846

- Queiroz, M. V. (2011). Rheumatic Diseases. Guide and exercises for patients. Lisboa. Lidel.
- Silvia Poliana Guedes Alcoforado, C., Araujo, C. F. d., Ramos, T. S., P.Urquiza, & Cantilino, A. (2022). Psychiatric Manifestations in Rheumatology. *Revista Debates Em Psiquiatria.* https://doi.org/10.25118/2763-9037.2022.v12.279

•

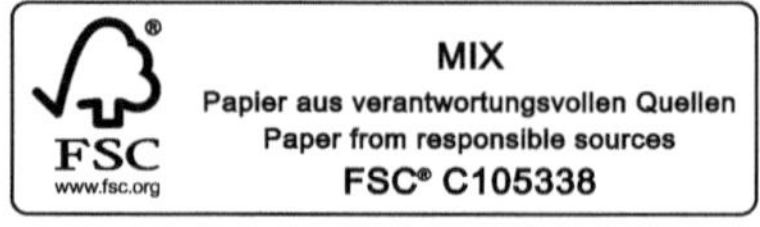


Printed by Books on Demand GmbH, Norderstedt / Germany